Detox Diet: The Way to Rejuvenate the Body

How to Lose Weight and Increase Longevity

By: Amy Zulpa

TABLE OF CONTENTS

Publishers Notes

Disclaimer

This publication is intended to provide helpful and informative material. It is not intended to diagnose, treat, cure, or prevent any health problem or condition, nor is intended to replace the advice of a physician. No action should be taken solely on the contents of this book. Always consult your physician or qualified health-care professional on any matters regarding your health and before adopting any suggestions in this book or drawing inferences from it.

The author and publisher specifically disclaim all responsibility for any liability, loss or risk, personal or otherwise, which is incurred as a consequence, directly or indirectly, from the use or application of any contents of this book.

Any and all product names referenced within this book are the trademarks of their respective owners. None of these owners have sponsored, authorized, endorsed, or approved this book.

Always read all information provided by the manufacturers' product labels before using their products. The author and publisher are not responsible for claims made by manufacturers.

Manufactured in the United States of America

DEDICATION

This book is dedicated to my dear friend Cassandra. She always had the right solution.

Chapter 1- What Is a Detox Diet?

People that want to look and feel as good as possible will find try to find a diet that will suit them. There are many of them that they can choose from. One of the diets that many people are interested in is the detox diet. The detox diet helps them to purify their system. When they want to do this, they will want to make sure that they understand the aspects of the diet before they begin it.

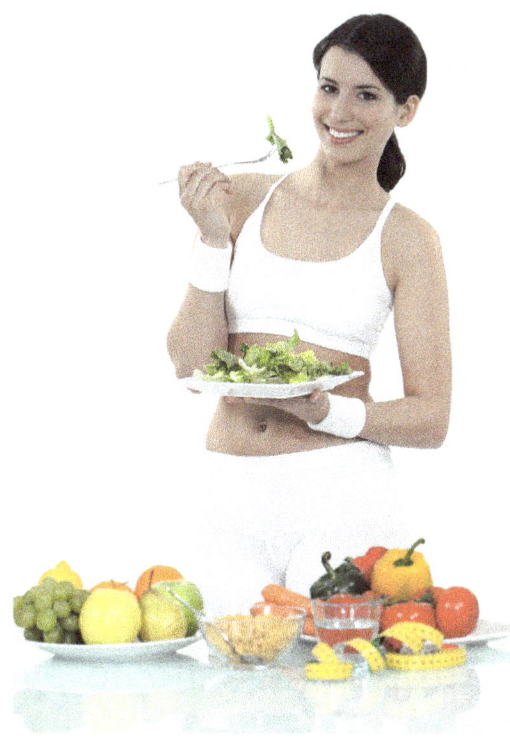

What Is A Detox Diet?

The detox diet is a way to cleanse the body of impurities. Many people like to do this in order to feel better. They should begin by cutting out coffee and sugars first of all. This will eliminate a lot of the reactions that might include headaches and other body aches when a person proceeds further into the detox diet. They should prepare themselves and get used to the lack of caffeine and sugar in their diet so that it is not a shock to their system.

Foods to Eat On the Detox Diet

When a person wants to begin the detox diet, they will want to have plenty of fresh fruits and vegetables in their daily meals. Fresh fruits are the best, but frozen fruits are acceptable too. Peaches, pears, pineapples and other fruits are tasty and good for the body. Raisins, dates and cranberries are also dried fruits that are particularly good for this diet. Vegetables that people will want to include in their detox diet are beets, onions, garlic, cauliflower, broccoli, artichokes and all different types of dark, leafy vegetables. These will help to nourish the body while detoxifying it of impurities.

Things to Avoid On the Detox Diet

There are all types of foods to avoid when a person is on a detox diet. It is important that a person give up dairy products and eggs when they begin to detoxify. They should avoid cheeses, milk, yogurt, ice cream, real butter and sour cream. It is also important that they avoid wheat products like pasta and bread. They will need to cut out sweeteners and gluten. Another thing that they must avoid is soy products and caffeine. They should also to avoid eating corn because it can disrupt the digestive system. They should notice a tremendous difference in the way they feel in about 7 days when they avoid these types of food products.

They Should Notice a Surge in Their Energy Levels in the First Week

When someone takes the detox diet seriously, they will usually notice an increase in their exercise levels in the first week. They will feel better and have a better frame of mind. As they continue with the diet into the first month, they will notice a great change in their body too. They need to stop the diet after a month so that they can get the benefits of the items that they removed from their diet. They should only eat those items on a periodic basis to retain their energy levels.

Exercise Is Important When a Person Is On a Detox Diet

A person that is on a detox diet should remember to keep up their normal exercise routine. They should exercise approximately three times a week. It should be around an hour of time each session, but they should not overdue it. Walking, yoga, dancing and other types of exercise will allow them to get a workout without overdoing it. During their exercise routine, whichever they choose to do, they should remember to keep themselves hydrated by drinking plenty of water. They should always have a water bottle when they are exercising to replenish themselves.

If It Helps To Get a Friend Involved, Then That Is a Good Idea

For some people it is difficult to follow any kind of diet without the support of another person. For this reason, is nice to have a friend perform the detox diet with them. They can consult each other on their progress, and help each other with their exercising. Having someone else involved in the process can keep someone in a good frame of mind too. It will make a difference when they know that someone else cares about what they are doing for their health.

People Should Use the Detox Diet Periodically

People should not use the detox diet on a regular basis. They should only do so periodically. They might want to do it every six months or once a year. If they do the diet too often it will not have the positive effects that it could if they do it periodically. It might cause them to become ill or lethargic if they diet in this way too often.

If They Have a Problem with the Detox Diet, a Person Should Contact Their Doctor

If they notice anything that seems out of the ordinary with their health or the way they feel, they should consult their doctor. If they notice very odd symptoms, they will want to get the help they need. They might be overdoing the detox diet, and they should make sure that they take the proper steps to correct the problem.

It is always a good idea to detox the body periodically. It is not a good idea to do so too often. People need to gain nutrients from what they eat on a daily basis, so they should make sure that they watch how often they do the detox diet to gain the most benefits.

Chapter 2- What Are the Real Benefits of Going on a Detox Diet?

Detox dieting is a hot weight loss phenomenon. Detox diets are designed to assist in fast weight loss and to cleanse the internal organs. Exactly what benefits are offered by an effective detox diet?

A detox diet works to cleanse the body because it is a form of fasting. This particular form of fasting limits the intake of the detox dieter. Doing this allows the body to continue and increase its everyday detoxifying activity. Certain inclusions in the detox diet have their own individual benefits.

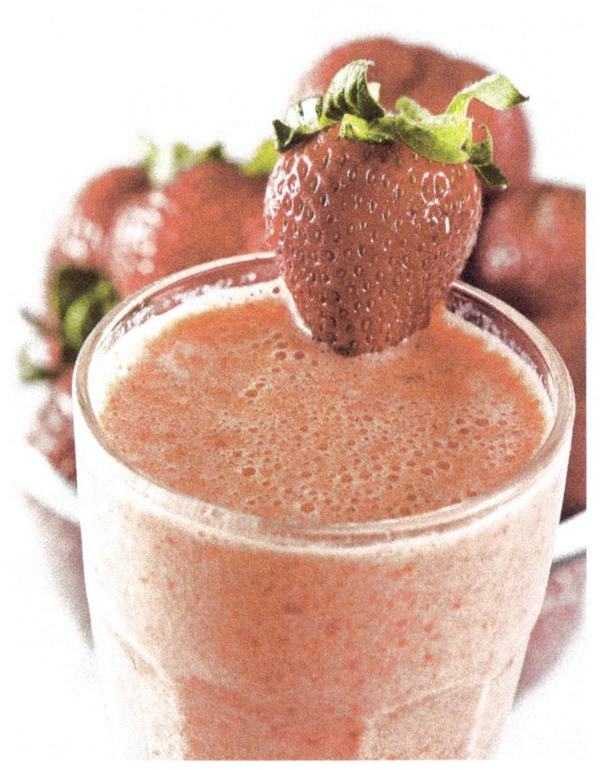

The first major component is liquid. It is usually water or water flavored with herbs, fruits, or vegetables. Drinking water every ninety minutes to two hours helps the dieter feel full and continually pushes toxins out of the system.

Some detox diets include brown rice. Brown rice is high in vitamin B. Vitamin B is known to reduce stress. It is also very high in fiber. High fiber foods help push toxins out of the system by promoting regular bowel movements.

Juice in a detox diet adds the benefit of preventing ketosis. Ketosis means that the body has no carbohydrates to burn for energy. The more energy a person has during a detox diet, the more they will want to move. Moving burns calories and will result in extra weight loss.

Eating less is known to extend the life cycle. This does not mean that a person should starve or become malnourished. It simply means that a person should eat a little less.

Embarking on a detox diet has a positive effect on the bowels, blood, skin, kidneys, and liver. A detox diet also has mental benefits as well.

The bowels eliminate toxins from our digestive system. Cleansing the bowels with a detox diet helps the body continue to eliminate toxins. Garlic is a common staple of many detox diets. It is believed that it fights harmful bacteria that are located in the colon. Cabbage is another helpful vegetable in a detox diet. It increases the elimination of potential carcinogens from the body.

Blood circulation is important to remove toxins from the body. Blood transports the toxins to organs for disposal. Many detox diets have inclusions of herbs, spices, fruits, or vegetables known for their blood purification. Brown seaweed is a good example of this. It is believed that brown seaweed acts as a natural blood thinner.

Skin is more than just something the outside world sees. Our skin is an organ. We release toxins through our sweat. We actually lose more toxins through sweating than we lose through our kidneys. It is important to choose a detox diet that incorporates ingredients known to rejuvenate skin. Pomegranates are thought to reduce the signs of skin aging by slowing down the weakening of the skin's collagen.

Our kidneys remove toxins from our blood. Those toxins exit the body through urination. Many detox diets use ingredients known for their diuretic effect to maximize the body's release of toxins. Almonds are great for detox. They can be used to make almond milk since cow's milk is not part of a detox diet. Almond milk is high in fiber and the good fats. They are also rich in many antioxidants that are believed to help ward off chronic diseases. Fennel is a vegetable that tastes a little bit like licorice. It acts as a diuretic and has only 14 calories for every half cup serving.

Our liver takes toxins and turns them into less destructive substances that the bowels and the kidneys can dispose of properly. A detox diet high in antioxidants helps the liver do its job in a more effective manner. Adding apples to a detox diet increases the intake of glucaric acid. Glucaric acid is known to help the body get rid of heavy metals. Ginger is another detox diet staple. For many people it works to reduce inflammation better than an over the counter pill; using a natural remedy instead of a pharmaceutical remedy benefits the liver. Parsley is also known to protect against liver problems.

Detox diets can make the dieter feel more alert and refreshed. Most people feel better about themselves when they lose weight. The important thing to remember is that some of the weight that is lost during a detox diet is water weight. Water weight loss can be maintained by staying hydrated even when a person is not participating in a detox diet. Detox diets make many people feel more energetic. Detox diets limit toxin intake while replenishing the nutrients our body's desire. This process can increase a person's mental focus. It is easier to concentrate when the body is not full of toxins.

A major benefit of a detox diet is that it jumpstarts a lifestyle change. Many people find that they enjoy the overall feeling of health they have directly after a detox diet. Some switch to eating raw foods or at least cut down on additives on a full time basis. This is a healthy lifestyle change that many people strive to achieve and fall short of using other diets.

It is important to consult with a health care professional before choosing a detox diet. While there are many benefits to a detox diet many foods can interact with medications. A doctor can discuss the specifics with the person interested in the detox diet. For example, we can consider the pomegranate. While pomegranate has many benefits and is thought to also lower the risk of heart disease, ingesting large amounts of pomegranate juice is not safe for people who take certain medications.

Chapter 3- How to Start the Detox Diet- Fasting

Before you consider the detox fasting diet, you must consult with your doctor. People of certain age groups are not advised to practice this diet. This includes people under the age of 18 or over the age of 69. Women who are pregnant or nursing are also not advised to do a detox diet. Other people not advised to go on a detox diet include those who are sick or recovering from an illness.

A detox diet is a special diet that focuses on the detoxification of the body. This diet would require you to consume certain foods and drinks. The foods consumed are wholesome. This includes frozen fruit, certain green vegetables such as broccoli and collard greens, grains, starches, walnuts, cashews, garlic, pumpkin seeds, split green and yellow peas, almond oil, and coconut oil just to name a few. Critics of the detox diet usually claim this diet to be unnecessary because the human body can naturally detoxify itself with the kidneys, the liver, the lungs, the colon, and the lymphatic system. The diet has proven to be more helpful than harmful to those who are generally healthy.

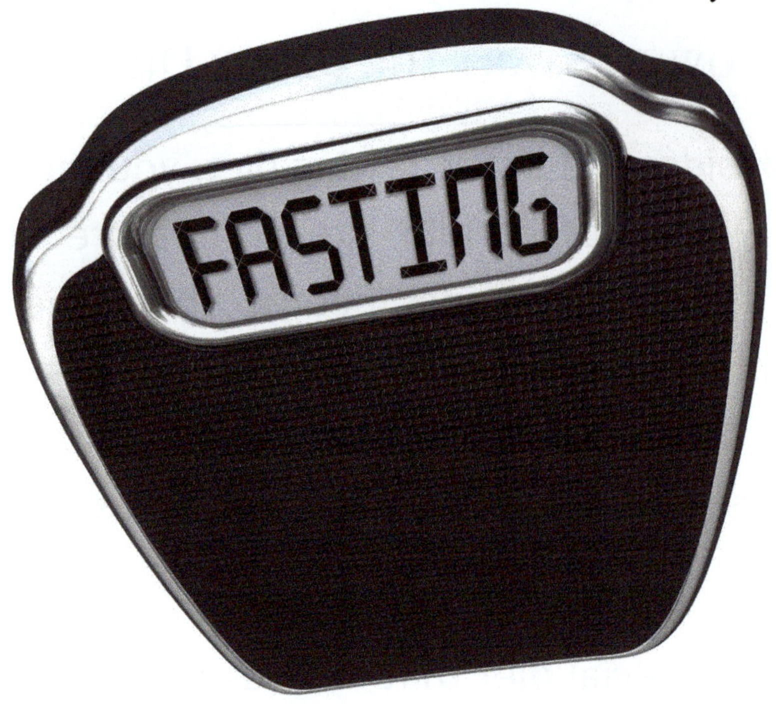

Fasting can be a part of the detox diet. It does not have to be biblical fasting because fasting itself has proven to be healthy, good for digestion, and great for detoxification. In a detox diet, fasting can vary over what you choose to consume and what you do not choose to consume. There are different types of detox fasting diets including juice fasting, water fasting, and fruit and vegetable fasting.

If you do not want to consume any solids while fasting, then consider juice or water diet. Juice fasting only requires you to consume juices that are all natural without any sugars added. Water fasting is the same. Fruit and vegetable fasting requires you to consume only certain fruits and certain vegetables prepared in particular ways. For example, fruits should be eaten frozen or dried when on this special kind of fasting diet.

Another consideration for the detox diet is deciding when and how long you want to fast. A good time to fast would be when it is quiet and there are no special events going on, such as weddings or birthdays. A few recommended lengths of time to fast would be two weeks, 7 to 10 days, or 2 or 3 days for beginners. Be sure to tell all of your friends and family when you are fasting so they know not to tempt you or invite you to an all-you-can-eat buffet.

If you are one who is really dedicated to practicing this special fasting diet, you can remove non-wholesome foods from your home. Be sure you stock up on supplies for the diet prior to starting it. Also, make sure you know what type of detox fasting diet you want to practice. Whether it is the juice, water, or fruit and vegetable fasting diet, be sure you are well prepared for it.

While dieting, be sure to do some light exercise such as a daily walk. Do not do anything too strenuous, for that can make you faint or collapse. If at some point during your fast you begin to feel faint or even dizzy, then you must end your fast. Keep in mind that when you end a fast you must not rush through the process. After completing or ending a fast you may feel like going to that all-you-can-eat buffet your friends invited you to. However, doing that after a detox can be harmful to your health. If you have completed or ended a water or juice fasting diet, then consider starting with fruits and vegetables.

Certain fasts have slightly different ways to be carried out in comparison to how a fast is usually and generally carried out. Juice fasting, for example, may require a different preparation process. Before starting a juice detox fasting diet you must prepare your body by increasing the consumption of vegetables. Rather than lasting for a couple of weeks, a juice fasting detox diet can last from 1 to 5 days. Also, the juices consumed are usually home-made using a juicer and mostly comprised of vegetables.

The water detox diet fasting also has some slight differences to its process. This includes gradually removing your usual intake of certain foods including sugar and caffeine and eating wholesome fruits and vegetables before starting the actual fasting process. The water detox fasting diet is also historically known to be the most common type of fasting both from a religious and healthy standpoint.

After completing this diet, your body will feel more cleansed. The detox fasting diet can improve the functioning of organs and tissues. Poisons, toxins, and even yeast can accumulate within the body. If not taken care of properly, the body itself may have trouble trying to naturally detoxify this buildup of toxins. The detox fasting diet will give your body greater strength and power to rid your body of and possibly prevent the accumulation of the poisons, toxins, and yeast. Getting rid of this accumulation can also prepare your body for weight loss. Whatever the reason may be, the detox fasting diet can be a healthy experience for you and your body.

Chapter 4- The Best Foods to Use for a Great Detox

As mentioned in brief beforehand certain foods are recommended for the detox diet. When you are dieting and trying to become healthy, it is necessary to detox your body. By getting rid of toxins and free radicals in the body, it is much easier to lose those excess pounds and become healthier. When doing a body detox, it is important to know what foods will help you achieve this.

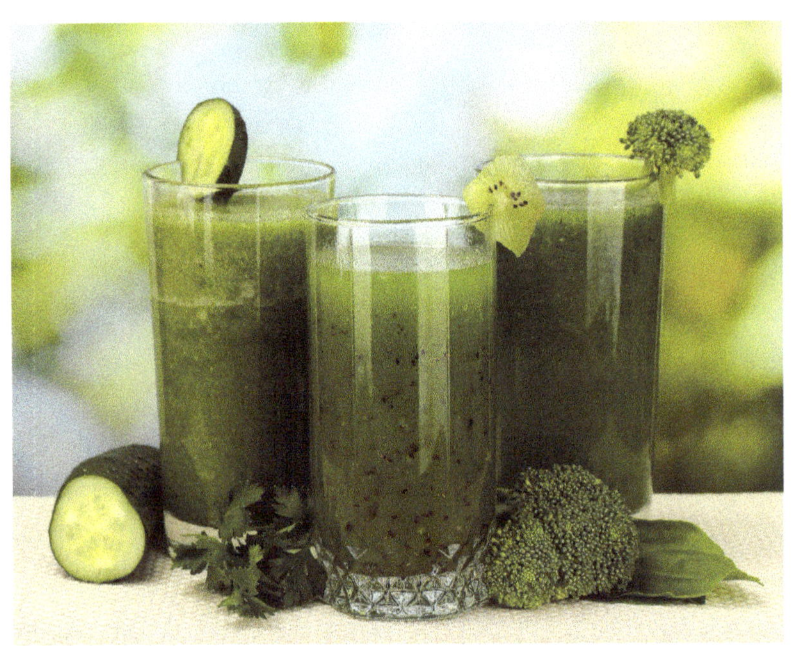

Artichokes

Artichokes are an excellent food for a body detox. They help improve your liver function. When your liver is functioning at its best, it produces more bile. This bile helps break down foods and allows the body to use the nutrients in them. The liver also helps your body get rid of anything it does need to survive. The artichoke is also filled with protein, potassium, and fiber that your body needs to stay healthy.

Avocados

For years, avocados did not get the respect that they deserved. Many people did not want to add avocados to their diets because they are high in fat. When people began to learn the difference between good fats and bad fats, avocados finally got the respect that it deserved as being a healthy and excellent body detox food. Because avocados are full of fiber and antioxidants, people are incorporating avocados in their everyday meals.

Broccoli

Broccoli is an amazing detox food. Not only is it filled with nutrients, it also works in the enzymes in your liver to turn the toxins in your body into something that is easily eliminated.

Broccoli is a very versatile food. You can add it into an omelet, a salad, eat it steamed, or mix it into a pasta dish. Broccoli can be incorporated into each meal.

Garlic

Garlic is known as a body detox super food. For starters, garlic will boost your immune system. Secondly, it will help boost liver function. The great thing about garlic is that your body will not develop a resistance to it.

Garlic can be used in many dishes; especially those detox foods that do not have much flavor. By adding garlic to those foods, you are making the dish taste better and giving your body detox plan a boost.

Grapefruit

Grapefruit is an excellent food for detoxing the body. When you eat a grapefruit, you are flooding the body with the fiber and nutrients that a grapefruit offers and at the same time it helps you remove the bad things in the body. It gives the toxins a one, two punch.

Grapefruit is also beneficial in weight loss. Grapefruit can help the liver to burn up fat. Studies have proven that grapefruit is an excellent diet tool.

Kale

Kale is an amazing super food that many people ignore. Kale can help to flush out the kidneys. Flushing out your kidneys is necessary during a body detox. Kale is so good that many doctors recommend adding kale in their diet when fighting kidney disease.

This vegetable is also packed with vitamins, minerals, antioxidants, and anti-inflammatory properties.

There are many ways to serve kale. It can be whipped into a smoothie, steamed, made into a soup, or added into a burger or omelet. With all of the ways to prepare kale, you will never get bored with it.

Lemons

Lemons are an excellent detoxifying tool. It is so well known for its detoxifying properties that there are several Lemon Detox Diets available. A lemon will flush the toxins from your body. It also helps with digestion.

Lemons can be used in many ways. It can be used over fish and in a salad. If you want a simpler solution, just add a lemon to water when you are drinking it. That is a great body detox option.

Olive Oil

Olive oil is the go to oil when it comes to cooking. It has less fat than the other oils available.

If you mix olive oil with fruit juice, it can trigger your liver to release its gallstones. If you are making a salad, try olive oil as a dressing. It will make your salad that much more healthy.

Water

Many people look past water when thinking of what to add to their detox diet because it is just too simple. When thinking of detox, many people go for the rare and complicated methods; however, water is one of the most important.

Water is responsible for flushing toxins out of the entire body. It also keeps the body hydrated which is very important. If you are not used to drinking a large amount of water, increase your water intake a little at a time. If you start drinking too much water too fast, your kidneys will not know what to do. You need to train your kidneys to handle a large amount of water.

Cabbage

Cabbage has recently become the main ingredient in the Cabbage Soup Detox fad diet. While you do not need to go to the extremes that the diet suggests, adding cabbage to your diet is excellent when trying to detox your body. Cabbage helps your liver by lowering your cholesterol. It also helps with bowel movements which help your expel toxins from your body.

There are many ways to incorporate cabbage into your diet. You can put it in a salad, a stew, or steam it as a side dish. There are also many slow cooker recipes available where cabbage is one of the main ingredients.

With all of the body detox foods out there, you should never get bored with your food when on a body detox diet.

Chapter 5- The Best Detox Diet to Cleanse the Kidneys and Liver

Before diving into any sort of specialized diet, you should be familiar with the process and know how you expect the diet to improve your health. The purpose of a detox diet is to cleanse the kidneys and liver. Detoxifying these organs will help your body better filter unwanted substances and operate at its optimal level.

Little do many know, but your body is constantly detecting, filtering, and disposing of toxins and poisons that seem benign to us. However, the purpose of the kidneys and liver is to detect what we can't discern, and rid the body of things that could potentially be harmful to it.

Completing a detoxifying diet to flush both the kidneys and live will improve and expedite the function of these vital organs. In addition, it will rid these organs of build-up that could be inhibiting their function.

The first step of the detox diet is to completely strike foods that will require your kidneys and liver to perform a good deal of work.

The first thing that must go is alcohol. Alcohol acts a bit like a poison when it enters the body and the kidneys and liver immediately work overtime to process the alarming substance that has entered the body.

The next thing that can absolutely not be a part of any detox diet is tobacco. Tobacco in any form is damaging too many aspects of both physical and mental health. The body can prompt a similar alert-like action to nicotine as it does to alcohol.

For optimal results, dairy should also be eliminated completely from your diet during the detox. Dairy is difficult for the body to digest. In fact, the majority of people in the world eat no dairy, and many eat extremely limited amounts of dairy.

Another important dietary restriction is sugar. Sugar includes not only regular forms of sugar, but any sweeteners, both artificial and natural (That means honey!). Sugars and sweeteners are loaded with fructose. Fructose can overload the liver, because the liver is only capable of processing small amounts of fructose at one time. In addition, our bodies have no physiological need for sugar, so we unnecessarily overload our livers when we consume sugars. Avoid added sugars and sugary drinks.

Along with sugar, grains should be avoided, or at least only consumed in small portions. Grains contain a great deal of sugars that can have the same effects upon the liver and the kidneys that sweeteners do. Other carbohydrates should also be eaten in moderation during the cleanse. The best possible cleanse would involve completely cutting carbohydrates from the diet, but this can be quite difficult for most people on a typical western diet.

Caffeine should be avoided as well. Caffeine can unnecessarily speed up the body and interfere with organ functions.

So what should you eat on the detox diet? Fruits and vegetables should become the staple of any detox diet. These foods should be consumed raw whenever possible. Cooked vegetables offer less nutritional benefits. Fresh is best. In addition, an adequate amount of protein should be consumed, though meats should be limited. Some of the best sources of protein that fit into a detox diet are legumes like lentils and beans. Ensure that you consume enough healthy fats while on the detox diet.

There are supplementary foods that can really enhance a detox diet and truly clean out and freshen the performance of the kidneys and the liver. Try adding artichokes to your diet. Artichokes contain a great deal of chemicals that are known to help rid the kidneys of toxins. Before meals, experiment with drinking a glass of apple-cider infused water. The acidity of the apple-cider can help your organs get rid of toxins before you add food to your body; giving them even more work to do. It's like a preventative measure before you have the opportunity to overload your organs. Similarly, drinking cranberry juice can also help your liver and kidneys rid themselves of unwanted toxins and waste.

A detox diet can be quite difficult to carry out. Most of us eat all of the restricted foods on a daily basis. It's hard to enact such a drastic change in diet, even if it is only for a short period of time. The best way to secure success is to pick a week to follow the detox diet plan that won't present many temptations or functions where you will feel obligated to partake of restricted foods. You'll want to avoid events like weddings, parties, or social gatherings where drinking or where the consumption of forbidden foods will be difficult to avoid.

While on the detox diet it is crucial to remember to drink adequate amounts of water. Water will not only keep you hydrated and feeling healthy, but drinking large quantities of water will actually help flush these organs of unwanted concentrations of toxins. This is particularly true for the kidneys. They require a good deal of water to function at their optimal potential.

Decide beforehand how long you'd like to stick to your detox diet. 1-2 weeks is typically enough time to begin to see positive results. Be sure to slowly transition back into your old lifestyle. Also note that when beginning and ending the detox diet, you may experience slightly abnormal changes such as atypical bowel movements and changes in food cravings and energy levels. This is normal. However, if strange symptoms persist, you should contact a health care professional.

Chapter 6- How to Include Supplements, Tea and Herbs in the Detox Diet

The New Year usually brings new diets, trends and exercise regimens. A popular trend amongst dieters is the detox diet. These diets are intended to rid and flush your system of impurities, so that you can resume a healthy eating habit. It is common to perform a detox diet prior to beginning your actual diet. This allows your body to reboot and start fresh.

Detox diets are a dime a dozen. They are extremely popular and quite successful if followed properly. They are specifically targeted at restarting and reinventing your system from improper eating habits, or bad food choices from the holidays.

They most effective way to kick off a detox diet, is to stock up on clear and healthy fluids. Water, tea, black coffee and lemon water are all ideal liquids to start detoxing. Water is one of the most important factors in maintaining a healthy body, and proper hydration. The more hydrated you are, the lower your body fat percentage will be. If you are interested in how to calculate your body fat percentage or hydration rate, you can purchase a scale that accounts for those measurements. Having a hydration percentage over 55 percent is looked at as properly hydrated. If you can drink as many ounces of water as your weight, then you are properly hydrating. For example, if you weigh 100 pounds, try to drink 100 ounces of water a day.

Drinking that much water a day may tend to become boring and repetitious. It is ok to mix up your liquids with natural supplements and herbal remedies. Local drug stores and grocery stores do carry a variety of detox teas. Detox teas are designed to help with the cleansing and purification process of your body. It directly will impact your liver, kidneys, blood and lungs. Most detox teas have various herbal and spices mixed in their ingredients. If you were to look at the listed ingredients of the teas you would see some of these most commonly used ingredients. They are cinnamon, ginger, fennel, sage, cloves, turmeric root, licorice and burdock root. A good detox tea brand to purchase is Yogi, as they offer many different kinds of detox teas.

Instead of purchasing a generic detox tea, try to recreate the ingredients and make one yourself.

Detox Tea

Ingredients

1 teaspoon of lemon juice
2 tablespoon apple cider vinegar
1½ cups water
1 teaspoon cinnamon

Directions

This is not a hot tea, but will resemble a cold mixed drink. Pour all the ingredients into the blender, and blend until all ingredients are liquefied thoroughly.

A more herbal dense hot tea can be made as follows:

Ingredients

2 ounces ginger root, peeled and sliced into thin pieces
1 cinnamon stick
2 cloves
Cayenne pepper to taste
1 teaspoon honey
½ lemon juice

Directions

Bring 12 ounces of water to a boil. Pour hot water into a tea cup and add all the aforementioned ingredients into the tea cup. Let the tea steep for 15 to 20 minutes. Add the honey and lemon juice once the tea has been fully steeped.

Another natural herbal detox tea that helps eliminate liver and kidney toxins is this dandelion detox tea.

Ingredients

6 tablespoons dried dandelion root
2 teaspoons lemon juice
12 tablespoons natural and fresh dandelion leaves

2 teaspoons honey

Directions

Bring a teapot to boiling water. Pour the water into your tea cup. Add the ingredients above and let steep for 10 minutes.

Along with incorporating herbals and spices into your regular detox diet, you can also include some natural supplements to help emphasize the detoxification process. Supplements are acceptable as they can aid and assist your body in gathering the proper nutrients it needs. Sometimes with a detox diet, you are not only cleansing the bad out of your body, but also the good. In ensuring a healthy detox diet, you need to make sure your body has the proper nutrients it needs to maintain normal daily functions.

There are many recommended dietary supplements that you can take while on a detox diet. Always take a daily multi vitamin, as it will provide you with the essential vitamins and minerals your body needs on a daily basis. A healthy supplement to invest in is turmeric. This herbal supplement is in the same family as ginger. This is a common supplement used in Chinese medicine, as it is believed to assist with digestion, reduce some arthritis aches and enhance liver functions.

Fish oil, whether you are on a detox diet or not, should be taken daily. Fish oil has been proven to reduce cardiovascular diseases. Fish oil contains the active ingredient, omega 3 fatty acids. This plays a role in sustaining and promoting mental health, improving cognitive functions, reducing the risks of diabetes and heart disease, and increasing your metabolism.

Another supplement that you can look to take while on the detox diet is milk thistle. It is a natural herbal supplement to help purify your liver. If you happened to binge drink the night before, this will help your body remove those toxins at a faster rate than your body would naturally perform the task. Milk thistle curbs liver disease, hangovers, recurring allergy symptoms and liver damage. Again, like fish oil, milk thistle is an excellent supplement that you are encouraged to take on a regular basis.

Most importantly, have fun with your detox diet. They are not only very successful with rapid results, but also a great way to restart your body, immune system and mind, and help create new healthy habits.

Chapter 7- Detoxing the Skin- The Best Methods

Whether you have embarrassing acne or a rash on your skin there are many healthy and efficient ways to detox the skin. Even if you don't have any visible things that frustrate you about your skin, detoxing will get rid of toxins, which are never good to have in your system. Toxins will make you feel sluggish and tired. By releasing them through detoxing, you'll find yourself feeling a bit more alive and energetic. There are copious amounts of ways to detox one's body, and finding the best method to go about doing so is incredibly important.

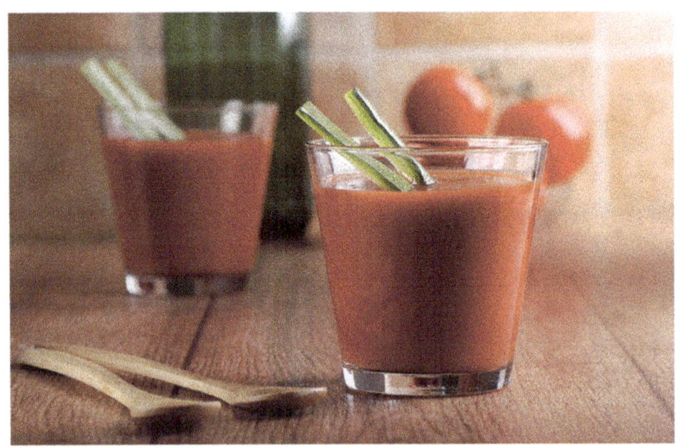

When it comes to detox, diet plays a large role in getting the toxins out of your body. When you eat brightly colored fruits and vegetables, you activate liver enzymes that help remove toxins from your body. This is done through the anti-oxidants found in those fruits and vegetables so grab some carrots or a banana. Now continuing on with your diet, always opt for organic foods. Limiting the foods high in pesticides and toxins will be extremely beneficial for you, while making you feel healthy and alive. Also, drink herbal teas. They will get your system working properly, while eliminating toxins from your body.

Having loads of toxins spread throughout your body is never fun, and if you want that clear and healthy skin you desire, a change in diet is going to be the best option for you in doing so. Stay off sugar. Yes, this means those sweet beverages that taste so good as you sip. But sugar is full of toxins that will slow your metabolism. You want to speed things up a bit, and by eliminating sugar, you'll be well on your way. Too much sugar will make you sluggish, and you simply can't afford that.

Instead of choosing drinks rich in sugar, opt for water. Drinking loads of water daily will help you get rid of toxins by sweating and urinating. The more you drink, the better your skin will look as you clear the system of the toxins that get in the way of its health. Try to drink about eight to twelve glasses of water a day, and begin to notice the difference in your skin, as water will clear out the nasty toxins. Another grand way to get rid of toxins in the body is by getting a massage.

Massages not only feel good and relaxing, but they also will help to improve blood flow throughout the body, as well as stimulating lymph nodes. So after your massage and properly hydrating yourself, a good bit of exercise goes a long way in getting rid of harmful toxins in the skin and body. Try to find a nice exercise routine that sees you getting about forty-five minutes of exercise daily. This can be done through things such as cycling, walking and jogging. Getting your daily exercise will increase the way you feel, and will get rid of toxins as you sweat them away.

When it comes to clearing away harmful toxins to the skin and body, it is important to kick bad eating habits and other dietary things. If you like having alcoholic drinks, work on eliminating that from your diet, or only having it in moderation if you must. Your diet plays a huge role in the amount of toxins in your body, and eating healthy will not only rid your body of such wastes, but also boos the levels of energy in the body and speed up that metabolism.

Along with the aforementioned options of fresh fruits and vegetables to consume, try foods that are rich in fiber. This will have tremendous benefits to your skin. Foods like oatmeal, nuts and whole wheat bread will do the trick. Adding fiber to your diet is easy and very beneficial. Some other food items to think about when wanting to clear your skin and body from harmful toxins, are homemade yogurts. Experiment with putting fresh fruit, honey, nuts and herbs to your diet. Foods like healthy yogurt that have good probiotic properties will help purify your skin from inside out. Now everybody loves a nice spa day, but they can get expensive and inconvenient at times. Bring the spa to your home with a nice facial treatment.

At home facial treatments may seem daunting, but they don't have to be. For example, for a healthy facial, try one in a relaxing spot at your home by doing a green face detox. The ingredients needed for the green face detox are as follows:

Ingredients

½ teaspoon of sea salt
½ teaspoon of white clay or green clay
A little green tea
A pan of steaming hot water
Skin detoxifying essential oils (eucalyptus, lavender, tea tree, etc)

Directions

After you have these ingredients, simply start out by exfoliating your skin. This is done by mixing your sea salt and the white or green clay with a little bit of green tea or water. This will make a paste in which you will rub into your skin. Allow it to sit there for a good two to three minutes, before rinsing with water and pat drying with a towel. Next, add whatever healthy skin oils you prefer, and steam the skin using the boiling hot pan of water. Do this for eight to ten minutes, getting rid of those skin toxins by purifying the pores. You can detoxify easily by eating healthy and changing your diet.

About the Author

For many years detox was a word that Amy Zulpa only associated with persons that were trying to kick a substance abuse habit. It was her friend Cassandra who introduced her to other forms of detox and introduced her to other aspects of detox. She learned quite quickly that is was beneficial to purge the body of toxins from time to time.

As Amy became more knowledgeable, she also learned that there were many reasons why people did detox. It may be that they want to purge the body to feel healthier; it may be that they are working on improving the exterior of the body like the hair and the skin. Amy found that a general detox and proper maintenance after did wonders both internally and externally.

www.ingramcontent.com/pod-product-compliance
Ingram Content Group UK Ltd.
Pitfield, Milton Keynes, MK11 3LW, UK
UKHW050841300726
14058UKWH00013BC/785

9 781631 876875